WALL PILATES FOR BEGINNERS

The Ultimate Guide to Strengthen Your Core, Improve Balance, and Enhance Posture with Wall Pilates

Copyright: © 2023 Ruth Gonzalez

TABLE OF CONTENTS

Introduction

Welcome to the world of Wall Pilates! In this book, you will go on a journey of self-discovery and physical transformation as you delve into the art of Pilates exercises designed exclusively for beginners.

Consider a world in which you may strengthen your core, improve your flexibility, and improve your general well-being while leveraging the support and stability of a wall. Wall Pilates is a novel approach to this famous training program, providing a safe and effective way for novices to enjoy the myriad advantages of Pilates.

Whether you are new to exercise or simply seeking for a new and inventive method to push your body, Wall Pilates is here to help. You will learn how to engage your muscles, improve your posture, and establish a strong mind-body connection through a series of carefully designed exercises.

This book is your entire guide to mastering the principles of Wall Pilates. From learning the fundamentals to gradually graduating to more complex techniques, you will have the knowledge and confidence to construct your own unique Wall Pilates practice.

So grab your mat, pick a wall, and prepare to begin on a transforming journey toward a stronger, more balanced, and healthier you. Allow the power of Wall Pilates to guide you to a new level of physical and emotional well-being.

WALL PILATES FOR BEGINNERS

CHAPTER 1

Benefits of Wall Pilates

Wall pilates is a variant on basic pilates exercises that combines the use of a wall for support and resistance. This type of training has various advantages for people of all fitness levels.

Improved core strength is one of the key advantages of wall pilates. Exercises against the wall involve abdominal muscle engagement, which helps to build and tone the core. This can result in improved posture, stability, and total body alignment.

wall pilates can assist increase flexibility and range of motion. The wall's support allows individuals to stretch their muscles safely and effectively, fostering increasing flexibility over time. This can be especially effective for people who have limited movement or tight muscles.

Another advantage of wall pilates is improved body awareness and balance. The use of the wall as a support allows individuals to focus on their body alignment and balance, which helps to enhance proprioception and coordination. This can be especially advantageous for older folks or those recuperating from trauma.

WALL PILATES FOR BEGINNERS

Furthermore, wall pilates can be a low-impact form of exercise that is easy on the joints. The wall's support decreases the amount of stress imposed on the joints, making it suited for people who have joint pain or injuries.

Finally, wall pilates can be a fun and challenging way to change up your training regimen. The use of the wall adds innovation and diversity to traditional pilates exercises, keeping your workouts fresh and engaging.

Overall, wall pilates has several benefits such as greater core strength, increased flexibility, higher body awareness, and low-impact training. It may be a terrific supplement to any exercise routine and can be tailored to individual requirements and skills.

CHAPTER 2

Getting Started: Preparing Your Space

It is critical to create a safe and comfortable setting before beginning your wall pilates exercise. Here are some tips to help you get your room ready:

Clear the area: Make sure you have enough space to move freely and safely. Remove any obstacles or furniture that may get in the way during your exercises. It's also a good idea to have a clear wall space where you can perform the exercises.

Examine the wall: Make sure the wall you'll be utilizing is solid and in good condition. Check for any loose or protruding things that could cause injury. If you are concerned about the stability of the wall, it is preferable to consult a specialist before beginning your practice.

Gather your equipment: Depending on the wall pilates exercises you intend to perform, you may require some equipment. A yoga mat or exercise mat for increased comfort, resistance bands, or tiny hand weights could be included. Have these items on hand before you begin your practice.

WALL PILATES FOR BEGINNERS

Dress comfortably: Wear clothes that allow for a complete range of motion and are easy to move in. Wearing anything too loose or baggy that could get snagged on the wall or equipment is not recommended.

Warm-up: It is critical to warm up your body before beginning your wall pilates program. Gentle stretching, modest cardio activities, or a short yoga sequence can all be included. Warming up helps your muscles and joints prepare for the forthcoming workout.

Maintain good form and technique: As with any exercise, maintaining proper form and technique is critical to avoiding injury and getting the most out of your wall pilates practice. If you're new to wall pilates, work with a trained instructor who can walk you through the proper alignment and techniques.

You may create an optimal setting for your wall pilates practice by following these procedures and carefully prepping your room. Always listen to your body and gradually raise the intensity and duration of your workouts.

CHAPTER 3

Essential Equipment for Wall Pilates

When doing Pilates against a wall, there are a few crucial items of equipment that can improve and assist your practice. Here are a few crucial points to consider:

Wall-mounted Pilates Bar: A long bar that is securely fastened to the wall at chest height. It offers stability and support for a variety of workouts, including standing leg work and arm movements. You can use the bar to engage your core and work on balance and alignment.

Resistance Bands: These elastic bands, which can be fixed to the wall and used for a variety of activities, are a great way to get in shape. They create resistance and aid in the strengthening and toning of muscles. Resistance bands are adaptable, allowing them to be utilized for both upper and lower body activities.

Yoga Mat: Any Pilates practice, even wall Pilates, requires a high-quality yoga mat. It cushions and supports your body during floor activities and helps to keep you from slipping.

Stability Ball: A stability ball can be used against a wall for core, balance, and stability workouts. It introduces insecurity, requiring your muscles to work harder to maintain equilibrium.

Foam Roller: For self-massage and myofascial release, use a foam roller against a wall. It aids in the release of muscle tension and the improvement of flexibility.

Pilates Ring: A Pilates ring, often known as a magic circle, can be positioned against a wall to give resistance and challenge to exercises. It focuses on the muscles of the arms, legs, and core.

Wall Anchor Straps: These straps can be fastened to the wall and utilized for stretching and strengthening activities. They give stability and support during motions.

CHAPTER 4

Basic Wall Pilates Exercises

Wall Squats

There are a few crucial elements to remember when performing Pilates wall squats. First, make sure you have a solid wall against which to lean. With your back to the wall and your feet hip-width apart, take a position. Slide down the wall slowly, bending your knees and lowering your body into a squat. Aim for parallel thighs, with your knees directly over your ankles. Hold for a few seconds, then slowly push back through your heels to return to the beginning position. Wall squats serve to build leg, glute, and core strength.

Wall Push-Ups

Wall Push-Ups are a modified variation of standard push-ups that are ideal for beginners or people who have inadequate upper-body power. Here's a step-by-step procedure:

1. Face a wall about an arm's length away.

2. Place your hands at shoulder height on the wall, little wider than shoulder width apart.
3. Lean forward and lower your chest on the wall, bending your elbows.
4. Return to the beginning posture while keeping your body straight.
5. Repeat till the required number of repetitions is reached.

Push-ups against a wall work your chest, shoulders, and triceps. Keep appropriate form in mind and gradually raise the challenge as you gain strength.

Wall Planks

Wall planks are a type of plank exercise that can be performed against a wall. Here's a step-by-step procedure:

1. Face a wall with your hands at shoulder height and slightly wider than shoulder-width apart.
2. Take a step back and stretch your arms, leaning forward until your torso is parallel to the ground.
3. Pull your belly button towards your spine to use your core muscles.
4. Maintain a straight body and keep this position for a set amount of time, such as 30 seconds to begin.
5. As you gain strength, gradually increase the duration.

WALL PILATES FOR BEGINNERS

Wall planks focus on your core muscles, which include your abs, back, and shoulders. Maintain excellent form and steady breathing throughout the activity.

CHAPTER 5

Intermediate Wall Pilates Exercises

Intermediate Wall Pilates Exercises are an excellent system to advance your Pilates practice and challenge your body. These exercises progress from the foundational movements of freshman- position Pilates to a advanced position of strength, stability, and control.

Wall Lunges

To perform Wall Lunges Pilates, follow these steps:

1. Stand facing a wall with your bases hip- range piecemeal.
2. Place your hands on the wall at shoulder height for support.
3. Take a step back with your right bottom, keeping your toes pointing forward.
4. Bend your left knee, lowering your body towards the ground, while keeping your right leg straight.
5. Push through your left heel to return to the starting position.
6. Repeat the movement for the asked number of reiterations, also switch sides.   Flash back to

maintain proper form throughout the exercise. Keep your casket lifted, core engaged, and knees aligned with your toes. It's important to hear to your body and start with a comfortable range of stir, gradationally adding the depth of the jab as you come more comfortable and stronger.

Wall Bridges

To perform Wall Bridges Pilates, follow these steps:

1. Lie on your back with your feet flat against the wall, knees bent, and arms by your sides.
2. Push your feet into the wall and engage your core.
3. Raise your hips off the ground, making a straight line from your knees to your shoulders.
4. Hold the bridge posture for a few seconds, focusing on squeezing your glutes.
5. Slowly drop your hips back to the ground.
6. Repeat the movement for the appropriate amount of repetitions.

Maintain good form throughout the exercise. Maintain a tight core, prevent arching your back, and elevate your hips with your glutes.

Wall Leg Lifts

WALL PILATES FOR BEGINNERS

1. Begin by resting on your back, hips near to a wall. Extend your legs, keeping them straight and together, against the wall.
2. For support, place your hands by your sides, palms down.
3. Draw your navel towards your spine to engage your core muscles.
4. Lower one leg slowly towards the floor, keeping it straight and in contact with the wall.
5. Exhale as you use your core and leg muscles to bring the leg back up to the starting position.
6. Do the same thing with the opposite leg.
7. Aim for 10-15 reps on each leg, increasing the number gradually as you gain strength.

Keep appropriate form in mind throughout the exercise.

WALL PILATES FOR BEGINNERS

CHAPTER 6

Advanced Wall Pilates Exercises

Wall Handstands

Pilates wall handstands are a tough but rewarding workout that improves upper body strength, core stability, and balance. Follow these steps to perform a Wall Handstand:

1. Locate a free wall space that allows your body to fully expand.
2. Stand approximately an arm's length away from the wall, facing it.
3. Place your hands shoulder-width apart on the floor, fingers extended wide.
4. Take a step back with one foot, then the other, until your body forms an inverted "V" shape.
5. Move your feet slowly up the wall, keeping your core engaged and your weight properly distributed.
6. Straighten your legs and arrange your body into a straight line once your feet are against the wall.
7. Firmly press your hands into the ground, using your shoulder and arm muscles.
8. Hold the position for as long as you can, starting with 30 seconds and gradually increasing the time.

9. To descend, slowly walk your feet down the wall while keeping control and stability.

Wall Pike Ups

Wall Pike Ups are a difficult Pilates exercise that strengthens the core, shoulders, and upper body. Follow these steps to execute Wall Pike Ups:

1. Locate a free wall space that allows your body to fully expand.
2. Stand approximately an arm's length away from the wall, facing it.
3. Place your hands shoulder-width apart on the floor, fingers extended wide.
4. Take a step back with one foot, then the other, until your body forms an inverted "V" shape.
5. Keeping your legs straight, engage your core and carefully walk your feet up the wall.
6. Shift your weight forward onto your hands once your feet are against the wall.
7. Pike your body and slowly elevate your hips, putting your legs closer to the wall.
8. Maintain your core engagement and thrust through your hands to lift your hips as high as possible.
9. Hold the pike position for a few seconds before lowering your hips to the beginning position.
10. Repeat the exercise as many times as necessary.

Wall Scissor Kicks

Wall Scissor Kicks is a Pilates exercise that focuses on the abdominal muscles, specifically the lower abs. Here's a step-by-step breakdown on how to do Wall Scissor Kicks:

1. Begin by lying on your back and extending your legs against a wall. Your body should be in a straight line, with your arms at your sides.
2. Draw your navel towards your spine to engage your core muscles. This will aid in pelvic stability and lower back protection.
3. Lower one leg slowly to the floor, maintaining the other leg against the wall. Maintain control and avoid making any unexpected moves.
4. Exhale and utilize your core muscles to bring one leg back up to the beginning position as you drop it. Rep this exercise with the opposite leg.
5. Maintain control and stability throughout the exercise by switching legs in a scissor-like motion.
6. Aim for 10-15 reps on each leg, or as many as you can complete comfortably while keeping perfect technique.

CHAPTER 7

Modifications and Progressions

Pilates, like any other fitness regimen, benefits from modifications and progressions. They enable people to personalize exercises to their specific requirements and abilities, assuring safety and effectiveness.

Wall Scissor Kicks can be modified to match different fitness levels or to address physical restrictions. For example, if you have trouble keeping your legs straight against the wall, you can slightly bend your knees. The intensity of the exercise is reduced, making it more accessible to beginners or people with poor flexibility.

Progression, on the other hand, is a method of increasing the difficulty of an activity as you become stronger and more proficient. To strengthen the workout with Wall Scissor Kicks, increase the amount of repetitions or add ankle weights. Another progression is to execute the exercise with your arms extended overhead, which puts your core stability to the test.

It's critical to remember that changes and progressions should be made gradually and with good form.

CHAPTER 8

Creating a Wall Pilates Routine

Pilates is a low-impact exercise technique that emphasizes core strength, flexibility, and full body awareness. A Wall Pilates practice is a wonderful place to start if you're a novice looking to add Pilates into your exercise program. This chapter will help you through the process of developing a Wall Pilates practice designed exclusively for beginners.

Step 1: Gather Your Materials
A Wall Pilates exercise doesn't require much equipment, but the following materials will come in handy:
a blank wall
A yoga mat or a comfortable workout surface
a strong chair
(Optional) Pilates ball

Step 2: Stretching

Warming up your body is critical before beginning any training activity. For around 5 minutes, do some simple aerobic activities like jumping jacks or running in place to get your blood flowing and your muscles warmed up.

Step 3: Pilates on the Walls

Exercise 1: Roll-Down the Wall
With your back to the wall and your feet hip-width apart, take a position.
Inhale, then exhale while slowly rolling your spine down against the wall, one vertebra at a time, as far as your flexibility allows.
Exhale as you roll back up to the beginning position.
5-10 reps.
Wall Squats

Place your back to the wall and your feet hip-width apart.
Slid down the wall slowly, bending your knees to a 90-degree angle.
Hold for 10-15 seconds.
To stand back up, push through your heels.
5-10 reps.
Wall Angel is the third exercise.

With your back to the wall and your feet hip-width apart, take a position.
Engage your core muscles by pressing your lower back against the wall.
Raise your arms to shoulder level and bend your elbows at a 90-degree angle.
Extend your arms upwards while you slowly slide your arms up the wall.

WALL PILATES FOR BEGINNERS

Return your arms to their starting positions.
5-10 reps.

Workout 4: Wall Plank
Place your hands at shoulder height on the wall and take a step back until your body is in a straight line.
Hold this stance for 20-30 seconds while engaging your core.
As you get stronger, gradually increase your holding time.

Step 4: Relaxation

It is critical to cool down your body after finishing your Wall Pilates routine. Stretch your major muscle groups, including the hamstrings, quadriceps, hips, and shoulders, for a few minutes.

Step 5: Progression

Consider adding variations or utilizing a Pilates ball for some exercises as you get more familiar with them to increase the difficulty. Always pay attention to your body and progress to more advanced moves gradually.

Step 6: Maintaining Consistency

In Pilates, consistency is essential. Aim to do this workout 3-4 times per week to notice gradual gains in strength and flexibility.

Step 7: Seek Professional Help

Consider taking a class with a trained teacher if you're new to Pilates to guarantee you're employing proper form and technique.

Remember that Pilates is a holistic technique that takes time and effort to master. Take your time as a beginner, and keep appropriate form and breathing in mind throughout your program. You'll notice changes in your strength, posture, and overall well-being as time goes on.

CHAPTER 9

Tips for Proper Form and Technique

Pilates is a workout method that focuses on precision, control, and good form. When beginning a Wall Pilates practice as a beginner, it's critical to focus on form and technique to maximize the benefits and minimize the chance of injury. Here are some important pointers to remember when completing Wall Pilates exercises:

1. Keep Alignment

Pilates emphasizes alignment. When performing Wall Pilates movements, stand with your back to the wall and make sure your head, shoulders, spine, and hips are all in a straight line. Proper alignment allows you to engage the right muscles and avoids tension on your back and neck.

2. Involve Your Core

Pilates is all on engaging the core. Pull your navel towards your spine to stimulate your deep abdominal muscles before beginning any exercise.

Throughout the exercises, this engagement will give stability and support for your spine.

3. Mindful Breathing

Pilates includes breathing exercises. To prepare for a movement, inhale deeply through your nose and exhale fully through your mouth. The breath should be controlled and synced with your actions to assist you in remaining centered and connected to your core.

4. Begin with the Fundamentals

As a novice, it is critical to begin with the fundamental exercises. The Wall Roll-Down, Wall Squats, Wall Angels, and Wall Plank are all great places to start. Master these exercises before on to more difficult variations.

5. Concentrate on Control

Pilates emphasizes controlled movements over speed. Each exercise should be done slowly and thoughtfully. Avoid using momentum to finish the exercise because it can jeopardize your form and efficacy. Slow and controlled movements more effectively engage the muscles.

Mind-Body Connection No. 6

Body awareness is one of the fundamental elements of Pilates. Pay attention to how each action feels and how it engages your muscles. This attentiveness allows you to enhance your form and engage the right muscles.

7. Make Good Use of Props

Props such as a Pilates ball can provide additional support and diversity. When utilizing props, make sure they add to the activity rather than detract from it. Squeezing a Pilates ball between your knees, for example, can be utilized to add challenge to the Wall Squat exercise.

8. Pay Attention to Your Body

Take note of how your body feels during the workouts. Stop the activity immediately if you suffer pain or discomfort that goes beyond the typical "good burn" sensation. It is critical not to push through pain. If you have any concerns, speak with a fitness expert or a healthcare physician.

9. Check Your Alignment on a Regular Basis

While doing Wall Pilates movements, verify your alignment by looking in the mirror or asking a friend. Because proper alignment is not always apparent, external feedback can be quite beneficial.

10. Progression Gradually

Consider raising your repetitions, extending your hold times, or exploring more difficult exercises as your strength and confidence grow. Make modifications gradually, however, to avoid overexertion or injury.

11. Consistency and patience

Pilates is a journey, and improvement may be slow at first. Maintain consistency in your practice and be patient with yourself. As you improve your form and technique, you'll get the many advantages of Wall Pilates, such as increased core strength, flexibility, and posture.

Finally, appropriate form and technique are critical for a successful Wall Pilates program, especially as a beginner. The emphasis on alignment, core engagement, regulated movements, and focused breathing establishes the groundwork for a safe and effective practice. Wall Pilates will help you build a strong, balanced, and resilient physique with time and dedication.

CHAPTER 10

Common Mistakes to Avoid

When novices begin a Wall Pilates regimen, they may make certain typical errors that might reduce the efficiency of their workouts and potentially lead to injury. Here are some frequent mistakes to avoid in order to maintain a safe and fruitful practice:

Inadequate Warm-Up: Skipping a warm-up is a common mistake. To enhance blood flow and prevent injury, prepare your body with light aerobic or dynamic stretching.

Incorrect Posture and Alignment: Poor posture and alignment can diminish the effectiveness of exercises and even cause discomfort or injury. When using the wall, always keep your head, shoulders, spine, and hips in good alignment.

Overarching the Back: Avoid arching your back excessively when practicing Wall Pilates. Keep your spine in a neutral position to avoid hurting your lower back.

Neglecting Core Engagement: Core engagement is fundamental to Pilates. Ineffective exercises can result from failing to activate your core muscles. Always keep your attention on your deep abdominal muscles.

Breathing Control: Breathing control is essential in Pilates. Holding your breath might cause tension and reduce the effectiveness of your movements. Remember to breathe mindfully and in sync with each exercise.

Using Momentum: It is a mistake to rush through workouts with momentum rather than controlled motions. Slow down and concentrate on precise, deliberate movements to recruit the appropriate muscles.

Ignoring Pain: Never ignore pain or discomfort. Stop immediately if a workout causes pain and talk with a professional to ensure you're not doing anything that could cause injury.

Overexertion: Beginners frequently overestimate their talents and overwork themselves. To avoid overexertion or muscular pain, Pilates requires gradual improvement.

Excessive Repetition: Excessive repetition without good form might cause muscular fatigue and damage your technique. In each exercise, prioritize quality above quantity.

WALL PILATES FOR BEGINNERS

Not Using Props appropriately: If you use props such as a Pilates ball, make sure you utilize them appropriately. Incorrect muscle engagement and instability can result from improper use of props.

Inadequate Recovery Time: It is critical to allow your body to recuperate. Overtraining without adequate rest can result in burnout and poor performance. Aim for a 48-hour recuperation period between strenuous sessions.

Comparing Yourself to Others: Try not to compare your progress to that of others. Each person's fitness path is unique, and it's more vital to focus on your own progress and accomplishments.

Neglecting Flexibility: While Pilates is great for strength, don't forget about flexibility. In order to balance your practice, incorporate stretching and mobility exercises into your program.

Skipping Cool Down: Just as you should warm up, you should cool down properly. It aids in the recovery of your body and minimizes the likelihood of muscular soreness.

As a novice, you can assure a safer and more effective Wall Pilates program by being aware of these frequent pitfalls and actively striving to prevent them. Proper form, technique, and patience are essential for obtaining the full advantages of Pilates while avoiding injury.

37

CHAPTER II

Frequently Asked Questions

1. What exactly is Wall Pilates, and how does it differ from standard Pilates?

Wall Pilates is a type of Pilates that uses a wall for support and alignment. It includes workouts that use the wall as a stabilizing factor, making it appropriate for beginners who may require additional support and coaching.

2. Is Wall Pilates appropriate for beginners?

Yes, Wall Pilates can be a great place to start for beginners. The wall provides additional support, making good alignment and technique easier to maintain. It's a safe and effective technique to get people interested in Pilates.

3. Do I need any additional equipment as a beginner to do Wall Pilates?

While no special equipment is required, having a clear wall space, a yoga mat or cushioned surface, and, perhaps, a Pilates ball can improve your practice. These fundamentals are adequate to get started.

4. How frequently should I do Wall Pilates as a beginner?

Aim for three to four workouts per week. Pilates emphasizes consistency. You can progressively increase the duration and intensity of your workouts over time.

5. Are there any restrictions on age or fitness level for Wall Pilates beginners?

Wall Pilates is generally appropriate for people of all ages and fitness levels. However, if you have any medical concerns or physical restrictions, you should get the advice of a healthcare specialist or a certified Pilates instructor to ensure that it is safe for you.

6. Can Wall Pilates help you lose weight?

While Wall Pilates primarily focuses on core strength, flexibility, and posture, it may be included into a comprehensive exercise regimen that aids in weight management. Weight loss can be aided by combining it with aerobic exercise and a well-balanced diet.

7. What are some frequent rookie mistakes to avoid when beginning Wall Pilates?

Poor posture, ignoring core engagement, leveraging momentum, and overexerting yourself are all common faults. Remember to use good form and technique, as stated before in this discussion.

8. Is it required to take Wall Pilates courses with an instructor, or can a novice practice at home?

While practicing at home is possible, it is strongly advised, particularly for beginners, to begin with sessions guided by a trained instructor. They can advise you on good technique, alignment, and progression, allowing you to get the most out of your practice while reducing your chance of injury.

9. Is it possible to mix Wall Pilates with other forms of exercise?

Absolutely. Wall Pilates is frequently incorporated into people's overall exercise routines. When combined with cardio, strength training, and flexibility exercises, it can provide a well-rounded approach to fitness.

10. How long does it take for a novice to experience improvements from Wall Pilates?

The time it takes for results to appear varies from person to person. Within a few weeks of consistent practice, you should notice gains in core strength, flexibility, and posture. Patience and constancy are essential.

11. Are there any workouts for beginners that target specific areas, such as the abs or lower back?

Yes, exercises such as wall squats and wall planks target the core muscles, while wall roll-downs and wall angels can help improve posture and spinal flexibility. Exercises to target specific areas might be guided by a professional instructor.

12. What should I wear as a novice for Wall Pilates?

Wear gym clothes that are comfortable and breathable, and that allow you a full range of motion. Form-fitting clothing can aid the instructor's or your own observation of your alignment and form during the exercises.

These frequently asked questions and their answers should get you started on your Wall Pilates journey as a beginner.

Conclusion and Next Steps

As you embark on your Wall Pilates journey as a beginner, imagine yourself in a story of transformation, much like the tale of a fledgling bird learning to spread its wings. Wall Pilates is your nurturing nest, providing a secure foundation for your growth. You've learned the basics, avoided common pitfalls, and gained insights into the world of mindful movement.

Just like our young bird, you have to start small, focusing on proper form and technique. You've made strides in building your core strength, flexibility, and body awareness. Your story is one of patience and persistence, and the journey has only just begun.

Next Steps:

Now, with your newfound knowledge, the story takes an exciting turn. Your next steps are filled with opportunities for growth and exploration. Here's where your journey continues:

Dive Deeper: Continue to explore the world of Wall Pilates. Consider taking a class with a certified instructor who can guide you through more advanced exercises and variations.

WALL PILATES FOR BEGINNERS

Set Goals: Define your goals. Whether it's improved posture, enhanced core strength, or overall well-being, having clear objectives will keep your story on track.

Stay Consistent: Like the bird returning to its nest daily, maintain consistency in your Pilates practice. Commit to your routine and enjoy the gradual progress you make.

Seek Inspiration: Seek inspiration from your own progress and the stories of others who have journeyed before you. Success stories and the transformation of fellow beginners can motivate you to reach new heights.

Embrace Challenges: Just as our young bird faces storms and winds, you'll encounter challenges along the way. Embrace them as opportunities for growth and learning.

Be Mindful: Stay connected to your body and breath as you continue your Wall Pilates adventure. Mindfulness is your compass, guiding you through each movement.

Share Your Story: As your journey unfolds, share your experiences with friends and family. Encourage them to join you on your Wall Pilates adventure, creating a community of support and inspiration.

Your Wall Pilates story is one of self-discovery, strength, and transformation. As you take the next steps, remember that it's not just about the destination but the journey itself. Embrace every moment, every challenge, and every small victory. Your Wall Pilates journey is a captivating story in the making, and the future holds countless exciting chapters waiting to be written.

Thank you for Reading

www.ingramcontent.com/pod-product-compliance
Lightning Source LLC
Chambersburg PA
CBHW070742260726
48660CB00007B/2939